Keto Meal Plan for 30 Days

Smart (Ready-To-Go) Weight-Loss Meals for Saving Time and Budget

By Taylor Allen

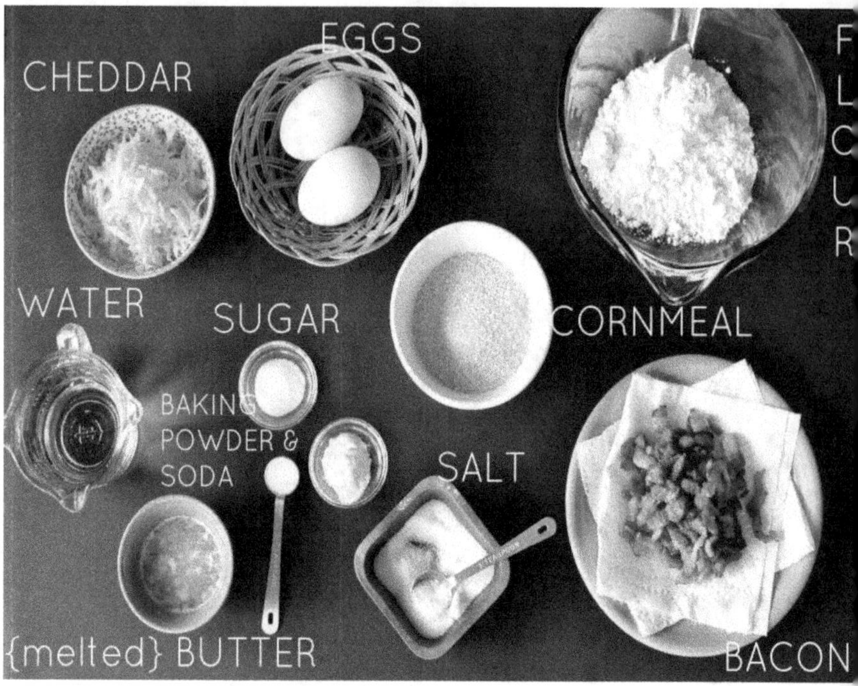

Table of Contents

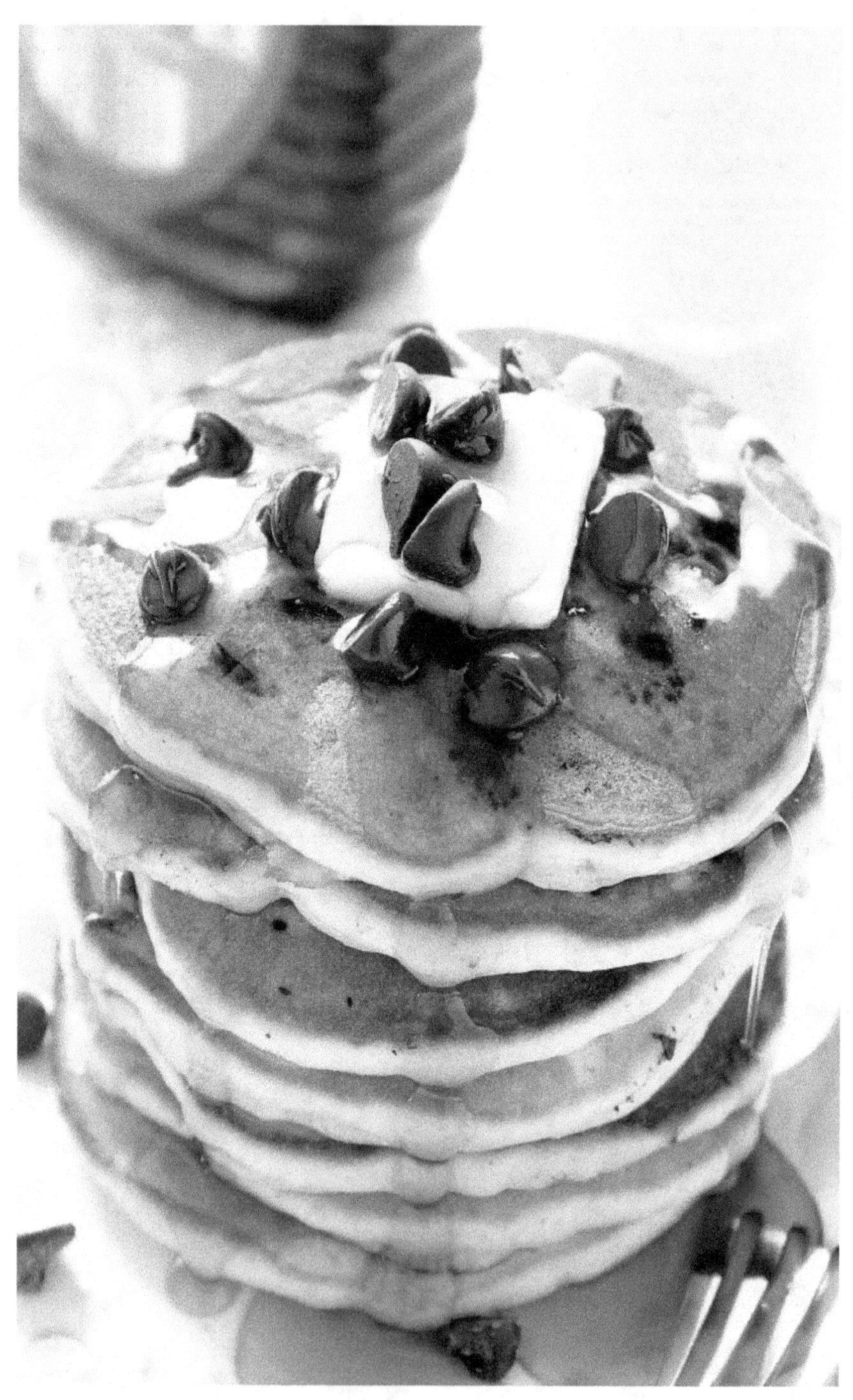

permission was gained from the owner. Any trademarks or brands found within arepurely used for clarification purposes and no owners are in anyway affiliated with this work.Any trademarks which are used are done so without consent and any use of the same does not imply consent or permission was gained from the owner. Any trademarks or brands found within are purely used for clarification purposes and no owners are in anyway affiliated with this work.

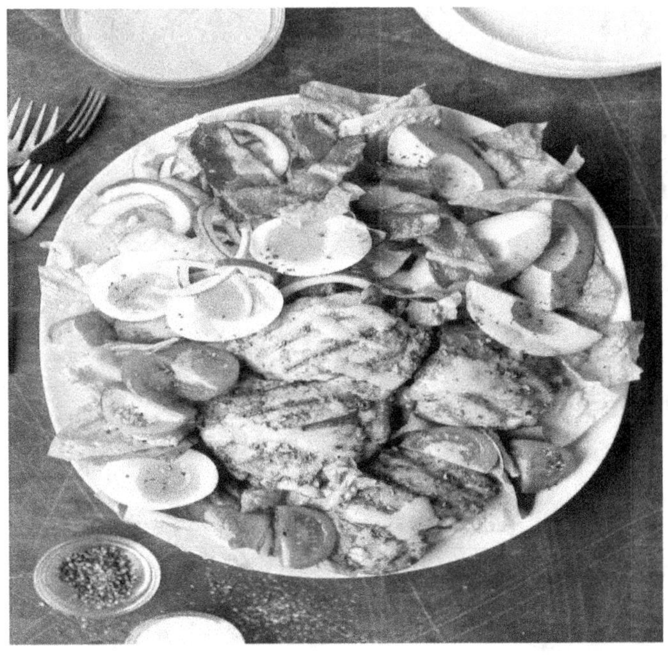

Introduction

Congratulations on purchasing your copy of "keto meal plan for 30 days". I'm delighted that you have chosen to take a new path using the keto meal plan to help your weight loss and prepare healthy meals to achieve your goal.

The keto diet is a low carbohydrates, which involves radically cutting down the number of carbs you consume and replacing them relatively high in fat food.

About the keto diet plan, it is advised to get over 75 percent of the daily Calories from fat, as well as the rest of their calories from protein. At the other diet makes up closer to 60% of daily calories, with protein accounting for nearer to 30 percent. Keto diet plan is an excellent tool for weight reduction. More to the point, it reduces risk factors such as diabetes, cardiovascular disorders, stroke, Alzheimer's, epilepsy, and much more.

Food prep is the most ideal approach to do so, plan your meals (even Snacks!), so you do not wind up reaching for a carbonated, carb-heavy food at a pinch. If it is possible to dedicate to a few hours each week on meal preparation, you will save hundreds of hours throughout the week on cooking, shopping, and choosing foods.

Meal planning Ensures you use whatever you purchase and makes it possible to adhere to the ketogenic diet plan. Successful meal prep demands some necessary equipment and essential ingredients like frying pan, knife, processor or blender, parchment papers, food containers.

Recipes in this publication will Supply you with an estimated preparation and cooking time, Amount of fluids, along with a listing of nutritional values including the internet Carbohydrates, fats, protein, and calories based on daily macronutrient amount.

 There are plenty of books on ketogenic meal plan, thanks again for choosing this book.

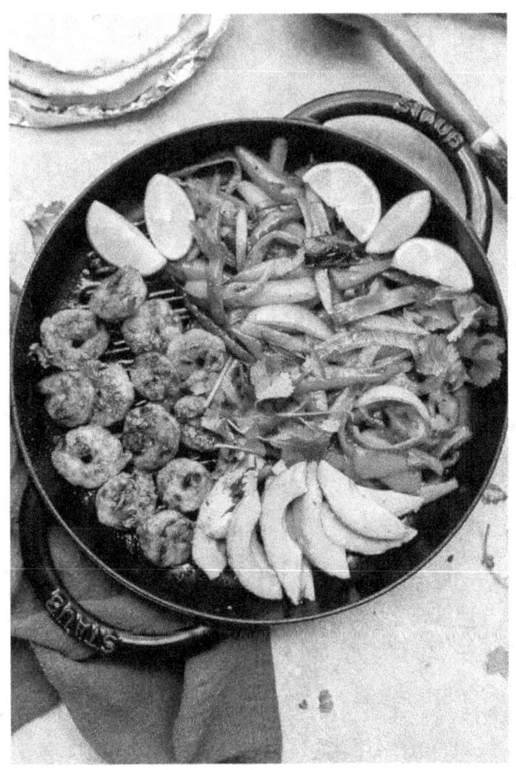

Chapter 1

Overview of keto diet

The ketogenic weight loss program is a high fat, low carbohydrate diet that places the human body ketosis. The slogan: "eat fat to burn off fat."

Weight loss is achieved by limiting carbohydrates and concentrating on food that high in fats. The traditional meal includes a four to one ratio of fat to each carbohydrates and proteins.

Today, the keto diet may be classified along with other high fat, low carbohydrates diet programs, like the Atkins or Paleo diets. Nevertheless, why these diets bluster advantages will most likely since they market ketosis. Consequently, in this manner, the ketogenic diet plan is not simply an eating routine," yet rather the foundation of those consuming regimens, alongside likewise the biochemical response which occurs when you practice the body of yours to eat fat for fuel rather compared to sugars.

While the Ketogenic diet has become famous for weight reduction, studies have also demonstrated numerous additional health benefits of adhering to a keto diet. As an example, a keto diet may help reverse adult-onset diabetes, and reduce symptoms of progressive mental disorders, autism, and atherosclerosis. In reality, the keto diet was first used in the 1920s as a natural remedy to stop seizures from epilepsy patients less a weight reduction diet.

Let's look closer at the way the ketogenic diet may work for dramatic weight Loss as well as it may improve your wellness.

How the diet works

The Objective of the keto diet for this to happen, you have to dispose of almost all starches from your eating routine arrangement.

Why? As per normal procedure, the body makes vitality from carbs, which can be put away as glycogen in your muscle tissues and liver. You spare adequate starches for around 24 hours of power. Today, the vast majority promptly renew our starch stores by eating vegetables, organic products, grains, and beans. Hence our carb "gas tanks" inconsistently secure decreased, and we continue consuming sugar for vitality.

In any case, if you genuinely can run low on sugar, your framework will switch gears and begin exchanging put away unsaturated fats into ketones, which might be used as an auxiliary power source. That is the reason the ketogenic diet is, in reality, compelling for thinning down.

Presently, in light of the fact that sugars are the human body's essential pick for power and fat is auxiliary, so the primary strategy to get your very own body to consume fat for fuel rather than starches is by putting your framework to a few" ketosis condition," normally by removing most by far of sugars from the eating routine arrangement. Without spared sugar, your body doesn't have any choice yet to dunk into your fat stores and begin changing over these unsaturated fats into ketones on the off chance that you require vitality. Enough fat could be spared in your framework to supply months (or possibly months) Value of imperativeness, which clarifies the motivation behind why individuals may endure fasting. The amount of fat that your body can use for vitality will be subject to your body cosmetics alongside the fat rate you are conveying.

Keeping up your framework in ketosis for broadened measures of time trains your body to consume fat for vitality better, and that is the way the keto diet plan can diminish your general fat without hungry because high-fat dinners keep you full more.

In any case, that the keto eating regimen won't cause weight lower, specifically on the off risk that you as of now have a base muscle to fat ratio. However weight reduction isn't the main bit of leeway or motivation to stick to a ketogenic diet plan. Give us a chance to investigate a couple of the extra included focal points.

Living the keto life

When you first get started on the ketogenic diet, your body isn't going to know what to think at first. The odds are high that you've been eating a lot of carbohydrates on the regular for quite some time, this means that your body has gotten really good at breaking down carbohydrates but, as a result, is a bit lax when it comes to using fat for energy instead. The smaller range of tools means that it will take your body longer to break down fat at first, leading to a feeling of sluggishness.

This feeling will be amplified thanks to new and different levels of insulin and glucose than your body is typically used to which will also lead to a general feeling of grogginess. Try and drink a gallon of water per day during this process as ketosis also purges electrolytes.

Secondary symptoms may include
- Dizziness
- Aggressive behavior
- Flu-like symptoms

- Issues concentrating

The most important thing to remember when dealing with these symptoms is that they are completely normal and to be expected. Knowing what to expect will make the first week pass more easily and before you know it your body will have entered ketosis and you will begin to feel better than you have in years.

The withdrawal symptoms may make it seem as though cutting down on your carbohydrates slowly might be a better choice. This is not the case, however, as ketosis will not start until your body has reached the target number of net carbohydrates per day for somewhere generally between 48 to 72 hours.

Once you are through the worst of it, you can start focusing on what you need to do in order to ensure you lose the most weight in the shortest period of time possible:

Types of keto diets

There are three different ways to adhere to a keto diet

1. Typical Ketogenic Diet:

This Typical ketogenic diet is among the much-investigated varieties of this keto diet. The SKD generally incorporates an eating regimen made out of five percent sugars, twenty percent protein, and seventy-five percent fat.

2. Directed Ketogenic Diet:

The concentrated ketogenic diet gives you a chance to include more starches around exercises, surpassing the Standard Ketogenic Diet five percent carbohydrates rule. This one could be a superior option for individuals that are amazingly occupied and train over twice every week. The most straightforward approach to discover when this is working for you will be to continue inspecting your ketone levels on the off chance that you include sugars after exercises and guarantee they don't show you out of ketosis.

3. Repetitive Ketogenic Diet:

This structure proceeds ketogenic times with high Carbohydrate days. It is commonly five ketogenic days, pursued intimately with two high starch times. Once in a while known as ketogenic sugar cycling, this variant of the keto diet on top carb days, the human framework will leave a state of ketosis. Notwithstanding, these "sugar refeeds" could be powerful for Muscle development contrasted with the focused on keto diet, since glycogen is The supplement which "packs" muscles Ketogenic carb cycling can likewise be said to be Not as a way of life stressor for various people, as the two high-carb days make The Repetitive Ketogenic Diet feel less prohibitive and simpler to pursue.

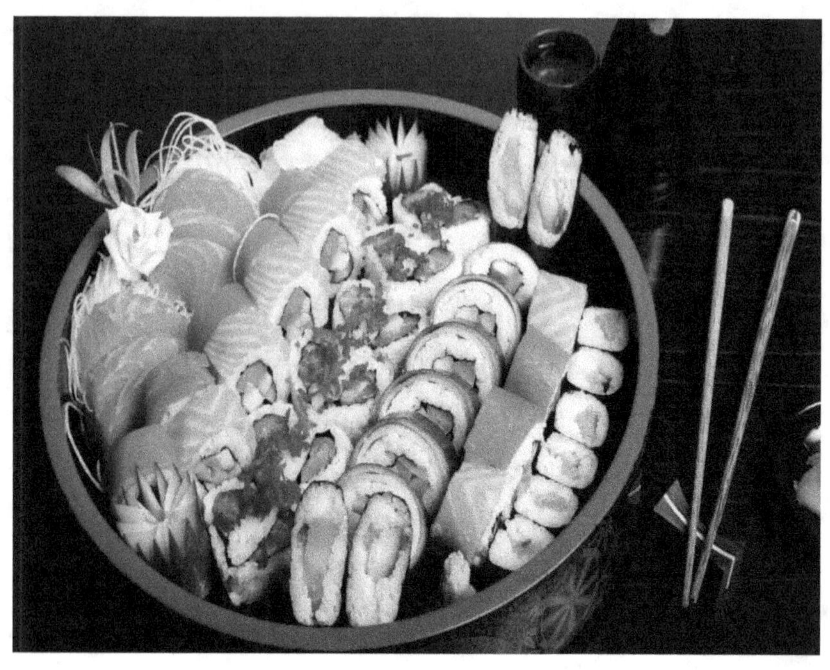

Advantages of a keto diet

Since the Keto diet evacuates all sugars and dull carbs, it can work as both a deterrent and remedial eating regimen for those in danger.

Keeps up Healthy Blood Glucose

If you build up a condition connected to blood glucose awkwardness, for example, type 2 diabetes, this implies your body has halted accurately reacting to insulin, and the hormone that pulls in sugar from your circulation system and into your cells to be put away and utilized as vitality. This is alluded to as insulin opposition.

There is Good and terrible news: While type 2 diabetes is for the most part expedited by overabundance refined sugar and starches in your eating routine arrangement, it's a condition that additionally can be turned around by changing the nourishments you eat. Once more, because the ketogenic diet evacuates most starches, it offers your body a chance to recharge and reset the speaking with insulin, which may upgrade insulin affectability and turn around blood glucose uneven characters.

At the point when pursued as an answer, ketosis can help improve other glucose conditions, including hypoglycemia and hyperglycemia. The authorization of social insurance proficient, the eating regimen May has pursued securely Long-term treatment for taking out sort two diabetes.

Improve Cognitive Function

The psyche can utilize two sorts of supplements for fuel: sugar, and ketones. This is in spite of a keto diet that can energize working. As a general rule, a few people today report improved the center, focus, and mental sharpness when they input ketosis.

The psychological exhibition might be because of the way that specific ketones, for example, hydroxybutyrate, make more vitality than glucose, which would genuinely make fat a progressively powerful fuel asset. There isn't much research to back this case up.

As expressed over, this keto diet likewise has been utilized proficiently for forestalling seizures in epileptic patients, especially the individuals who don't respond to the drug. While it isn't apparent how this technique functions, the examination shows disposing of fats and copying the effect of starvation may hinder the neuron stations that lead to the "electric tempest in the cerebrum" that outcomes in a seizure.

Additionally may furnish help Patients with disarranges - Alzheimer's infection. Research demonstrates that with the beginning of Alzheimer's, the synapses quit reacting to insulin, which irritates the mind. By confining carbs, the keto diet May help upgrade Insulin affectability when concerning blood glucose and cerebrum work.

Lift Skin Health

An eating routine that is high-crab was appeared to initiate oil generation, which is a wellspring of skin break out. Wiping out sugar from the eating regimen may help improve hot skin conditions, for example, psoriasis and dermatitis. The nutritious fats urged to the keto diet supply the structure squares of skin cells.

Hormonal Balance

The rest of your hormones may likewise lift and furthermore fix uneven hormonal characters, for example, polycystic ovarian disorder, or PCOS since ketosis can improve insulin capacities.

Research demonstrates that the keto diet may likewise improve the patient's response. One investigation announced an improvement in enthusiastic working and dozing in patients experiencing chemo that was following an eating routine.

Another way a keto diet can add to weight decrease is by adjusting. They top coincidental in parts, further prompting weight reduction since nourishments likewise are wealthier any longer satisfying than carbs.

Malignant tumorous use sugar as a wellspring of vitality to create. Therefore, by starving the cells, a keto diet is recommended to moderate tumor development in malignant growth patients in all stages.

Control Food Cravings

Another way a keto diet can realize weight reduction is by adjusting your glucose levels, which lessens desires for sugars. Since high-fat sustenance's are likewise more extravagant and considerably more satisfying than starches, they even top you off in short segments, further bringing about weight reduction.

Anticancer Properties

Malignant tumorous Use glucose as the essential Source of vitality to develop. For this a keto diet plan, Motive is recommended to moderate tumor Increase in malignancy Patients of all stages by starving the cells.

How to follow the keto diet

Since every individual has an alternate muscle to fat ratio percent and supplement requests, there isn't any one-estimate fits-all caloric or macronutrient rule for getting into ketosis.

By the method, for example, competitors who train a couple of times each week will even now have the option to go into a condition of ketosis by ingesting a greater extent of starches, in contrast with somebody who's generally stationary.

The quantity of sugars you're apportioned day by day and the best kind of keto diet for you to pursue relies upon your present weight, muscle to fat ratio percent, and stature, sex, and wellness and movement levels.

Guide to calculating macros for weight loss.

Determining your keto macros is the very first step you may take when beginning on a ketogenic diet plan.

However, until we jump to keto macros, let us quickly pay what macros are and their significance on keto.

What Are Macronutrients?

Macros are brief for macronutrients. They're classes of nutrients that give the human body. Energy is provided by some macronutrients. Others, like fiber and water, are required for different explanations. Within the following guide, we are going to be focusing on the three principal kinds that create electricity in the kind of calories. They're Fats, Carbs, and Proteins. Let us peek at how each of these works.

Proteins

Nails and your hair are made from protein. Your system uses protein to build and repair muscle cells. It is also the nutrient which produces hormones, enzymes, and other body chemicals. All whatsoever, protein is also a significant building block of bones, tendons, cartilage, muscles, skin, and even blood. However, that is not all there's to protein along with its physiological functions. Protein can also be instrumental in controlling your metabolism. It is the main reason it is recommended in weight reduction programs.

You can enhance your metabolism. Needless to state, it has an integral role in any healthful diet such as the ketogenic diet. Protein from animal resources is popular. However, you may get protein in the foods that are various. Protein can be determined in meat, fish, chicken, milk, nuts, seeds, legumes, as well as in vegetables which includes kale.

Carbohydrates

Carbohydrates are the meals villain Men and Women that are contemporary as it is the source of Like to hate. However, it is the macro Energy to the body. It's not an overstatement to mention that many people's bodies have been Operate by carbs. Carbohydrate assists fuel your mind, kidneys, muscles, heart, and Central nervous system. For Example, fiber is a Form of carbohydrate which aids Indigestion, providing you an awareness of fullness. It additionally helps to keep blood Cholesterol levels within the check. Carbohydrates are available in vegetables, grains, Fruits, seeds, nuts, and dairy goods.

Fats

Oils and fats would be macronutrient's kinds. They're also referred to as triglycerides and play a vital part of a healthful diet. Generally, fats constitute roughly 15-25percent of your overall calories in many diets. However, fats would be the essential macronutrient, which makes up to 60-75 percent of your caloric consumption up.

This is only because keto diets use this macro because the Main energy supply to construct ketone bodies. Fat can also be the most energy compact macro of providing nine calories a gram. That is more than twice the energy in contrast to protein and carbohydrates that provide four calories each gram. You can come across fats in items like nuts, seeds, olives, along with avocados. Unhealthy, artificial fats are most usually found in processed foods such as pizza.

What If Your Macros Be?

On any dietary plan, take a couple of different facets into consideration. Moreover, it begins with your daily calories. Naturally, so this is unique to you, and it is different for everyone. Things, for example, age, weight, activity level, and sex, influence your total calorie intake. Intuitively, even if you're busy, you'll need more calories a day. However, if you're attempting to eliminate weight, you might want to cut back your calorie intake. Once you've got this figure prepared, you can compute just how much fat, protein, and carbohydrate to eat. As a guideline, here would be the median macro parts of regular diets.

Alternatively, Government sources indicate 0.8 g of protein each g in kilograms. Your protein ought to be approximately 48 g should you consider 60kg.

Carbs: 50-70percent of daily calories. Taking the center, 60% are used by our macro calculator. Irrespective of your daily budget to your carbohydrates, limit your sugar consumption to 10 percent of your daily calories in the maximum. This guarantees that you maintain your foods balanced, healthy, clean, and wholesome.

Fats: fats 10-15percent of daily calories. Much like carbohydrate fats Come in the level of wellness degree. Adhere to healthy fats such as olive oil, olive oil, also fats that are inflammatory. Keep away from synthetic, saturated fats such as margarine and peppermint oils. Usually used soybean oil can also be prevented.

These macro parts must function as the beginning point in planning your Diet. You may also utilize the algorithmic calculator to compute your macronutrients. This way you may have a more precise figure.

Calculate your daily macros

1. Calculate maintenance calories:

Your body weight in (lbs) × (14 to 15) = maintenance calories per day

2. Calculate surplus calories

Subtract 500 calories from step one calculated answers (maintenance calories per   day – 500 calories) = surplus calories

3. Calculate protein:

Your bodyweight (lbs) × 1.0 = protein amount per day in grams

4. Calculate fat:

Your bodyweight (lbs) × 0.3 = fat amount per day in gram

5. Calculate carbs:

 (Remaining calories from step two) ÷ 4 = carbohydrate amount per day

Who Should Not Follow the Keto Diet?

The diet isn't suggested for the following:

1. Individuals with coronary disease or with no gallbladder, since fat is much more challenging to digest
2. Individuals who have experienced bariatric surgery (weight loss/gastric bypass) since carbohydrates are harder to consume
3. Women That Are nursing or pregnant, since protein demands are high.
4. Kids, since protein needs differ by age
5. People with pancreatic insufficiency, since fats are more challenging to digest
6. Individuals prone to kidney stones (possibly because of fluid and salt balance varies)
7. Individuals That Are naturally very lean because weight reduction may happen for a few
8. Individuals with anorexia.

Tips for success and mistakes to avoid

Start Small: An easy way to form a habit is to ease yourself into it. If you start out trying to run a marathon, you'll probably find it a bit difficult, may hurt yourself, and not see any benefits. Starting off your exercise habit with something small like a 10 minute walk will let you build up to the more intense activities.

Plan Ahead: This one ties into making a schedule and sticking to it, but expands upon it a bit more. Plan your week ahead of time with time set aside for your potential healthy eating habits. Planning several days ahead will make your schedule easier to follow.

Even planning a single day at a time is better than no plan. If you wake up and plan your day, you'll at the very least have a schedule set for the following 24 hours. A week is generally better because it does allow you to plan several days at a time without over planning (because planning a month is a bit much).

Know How to Deal with Ups and Downs: No matter how positive and motivated you are, there will be times when you don't want to work on being healthier. Motivation wears out, it's inevitable. That's why it's essential you make a habit of dealing with the highs and lows of your habit forming. You can counted the lows with several strategies. Having a group of peers, friends, or coworkers will help keep you motivated when your own motivation won't cut it.

Cope with the Lows of Habit Forming: In a weird meta-habit kind of way, it takes habits to form habits. It's important to make a habit of dealing with your less-than-motivational times.

As mentioned above, having a group of peers to help guide you, will keep you motivated and pushing through the tough times. Honestly, a lot of the previously mentioned habits can help pull you through the tough times with flying colors. Asking for help will inspire you, forming a group (contest or competitive) will give you a responsibility to someone other than yourself, etc. The most important habit is to get up and exercise as soon as your schedule dictates it. Without that sense of self motivation, the other habits will not be as easy to form.

Stay full, stay focused: While it is important to refrain from snacking as much as possible during the transition phase, it is even more important to prevent yourself from reaching a point where your hunger overtakes your ability to reason. This is because if you let your hunger reach a point where you are out of control it will be much less likely that what you put into your body is going to beneficial to your quest for ketosis. As it would only take a bag of chips or an order of French fries to push you out of ketosis for a day or two, it is better to stay away from the razor's edge whenever possible.

This can be easily prevented with a little preplanning, however, as it shouldn't take much extra effort to guarantee that you always have something keto-friendly on hand. Likewise, you are going to want to refrain from skipping whole meals entirely and try and make an effort to eat at the same time every day to ensure the transition proceeds as smoothly as possible. If you can get yourself into a routine early on, then your body will know what to expect and will be able to better control itself between meals.

Calories still matter: While following a keto diet means you need to be more worried about what goes into a meal than what its total caloric value is, this doesn't mean you are going to want to disregard calories entirely. While a given dish might have an ideal amount of fats, carbs and proteins, if a single serving weighs in at over a thousand calories that isn't a healthy option no matter how you look at it. Moderation is key to a healthy waistline, no matter what those calories are made up of. As such, make sure you understand what a healthy number of calories is for a person of your age, sex and exercise habits. Remember, just because you are making an effort to eat healthy doesn't mean there isn't more still for you to do.

Have the right foods on hand at the right time: When you are exercising regularly, it can be easy to get a little lax now and then when it comes to what you are eating exactly. However, if you use the fact that you exercise as an excuse to eat poorly, you will risk putting your ketogenic state at risk, canceling out all of your hard work as a result. What's more, you will find that your overall results will be much improved if you make it a point of keeping enough healthy fats in your system to power your entire workout. Likewise, you are going to want to follow up with exercise routine with extra protein to ensure your muscles have the tools they need to grow as a result.

Furthermore, while you will want to keep to a high-intensity workout in order to get into a ketogenic state as quickly as possible, once that is completed you may want to take it somewhat easier, especially if you know you won't be able to eat for a while after the fact. Studies show that a longer, milder period of exercise burns the same number of calories as a short, intense workout, while also leaving you less hungry as a result. As such, if you stick to a more moderate workout you are less likely to feel the need to binge after the fact.

Remember the three-color rule: When following the keto diet, there is no reason you should fail to experience as much variety in your day to day diet as anyone else. However, as with any new diet, early on it can be easy for you to find a handful of things that you like and stick with them, simply because finding new things to eat may seem intimidating. This is not recommended, however, as following the keto diet is more about building a new and improved healthy lifestyle, something that won't be possible if you never try anything new. As such, a good way of broadening your horizon is to eat something that is green, something that is red and something that is orange at every meal. Foods that are these colors tend to naturally be healthier and full of more filling nutritional content than the alternative. What's more, these foods are often credited with making those who eat them look and feel younger as well. This naturally aligns with the keto diet's benefits, supercharging them even more.

Stay hydrated: Remaining in a ketogenic state is naturally dehydrating which means that you are going to want to make a point of drinking more water than you normally do, especially if you tend to remain rather dehydrated normally. A good rule of thumb is that while you are in ketosis you are going to want to drink at least a gallon of water each day. While this may seem difficult at first, especially if you don't drink a lot of water regularly, you will be able to build up to it with practice and the results will likely surprise you. This isn't the only reason why a gallon a day should be your goal, as it will naturally help you to lose more weight than you otherwise would, simply because you will retain less water weight if you are well hydrated.

Watch your salt intake: While a vast majority of the recipes in the later chapters of this book leave it up to you how much salt you want to eat with your meal, early on at least it is important to keep your salt intake to a minimum. First and foremost, cutting down on the amount of salt that you eat will likely make you feel less hungry than you otherwise would, an especially important boon during the ketogenic transition phase. Consuming more than the recommended amount of salt each day has also been proven to make it more difficult to lose weight overall; so much so, that cutting out most of the salt from your diet has been known to result in a slimmer waistline in just three weeks.

Spice things up: After the worst of the keto flu has abated, if you still find yourself feeling hungry at the end of every meal, then your macros might not be to blame. Instead, you may be consuming less of the types of spices that generally help you body to know when it has had enough, leaving you feeling hungry despite the fact that you actually ate a full meal. Capsaicin spice, one of the most commonly used means of making food spicy, has the side effect of increasing the rate that endorphins are released from the body increasing the rate at which you feel full as a result. What's more, you can buy it as an additive and add a little bit of it to all of your meals, helping to train your body to your new way of eating more easily.

Keep a food journal: While early on it will likely feel that following the keto diet only means that you aren't allowed to eat anything that you used to enjoy, it is important to focus on the fact that this feeling won't last forever by actively proving to yourself that this is simply not the case. In order to help you get over this feeling as quickly as possible, you may find that creating a food journal is an effective step. Creating a food journal is easy, all you need to do is write down all the details about each meal you eat, including how the food was prepared, why you choose the meal in question, when and where you ate it and your overall thoughts on the meal itself. This will not only make it easier for you to find new things that you like, it will also help to ensure that you are sticking to your required macros as strictly as possible to ensure that you are actively making progress towards ketosis.

Before you get started it is best to keep in mind that your food journal is only going to be effective if you keep at it 24/7. A partially completed food journal is just a waste of time and won't do you any good. When you get started, go for broke and seriously commit yourself to the task at hand.

Eat at a more leisurely pace: During the transition period, in addition to having to deal with flu-like symptoms, you are likely going to be dealing with extreme hunger pangs that are really just a cover for your body's desire to stop having to work so hard and switch back to burning glucose for fuel. An easy way to counteract those feelings is to simply take longer to eat each of your meals. Eating faster certainly doesn't help you to feel full more quickly, as food can only move through your system so quickly. Instead, it actually makes you feel more hungry as it does not give your body the time it needs in order to realize that it is actually full.

To ensure that you get the full benefit from every meal, a good habit to get into is that of chewing each bite of food a full 10 times before you swallow. This will ensure that the correct signals have the time they need to get to where they need to go, helping you to feel full when you are actually full as a result.

Keep tabs on ghrelin: As noted previously, ghrelin is the hormone that causes your body to feel hungry which means that not paying attention to it is a great way to find yourself reaching for a snack full of carbs come the middle of the afternoon. The most reliable way to ensure its impact is as minimized as possible is to ensure that you have something healthy on hand to put into your body to keep the ghrelin gremlin at bay. This will ensure that your body is always in the middle of digesting something which means it won't be able to produce ghrelin at the same time. It is also important to keep in mind that the amount of time between meals that will maximize this effect is going to vary for everyone which means a bit of trial and error may be required.

Avoid skipping meals: While cutting down on your overall caloric intake is a great way to speed up the transition period as much as possible, this doesn't mean that you are going to want to go around skipping meals all together. Not only does skipping a meal cause your body to wonder where its next influx of calories is going to come from which can cause issues down the line. What's worse, it can lead to overeating which is a sure-fire way to push yourself out of ketosis and cause the whole process to take much longer than it otherwise would.

Not preparing properly: While the ketogenic diet is fairly easy to stick to overall, it doesn't naturally lend itself to spontaneous eating, at least in most parts of the world. As such, when you are heading out into the world, it is important to be prepared with your own snacks to ensure you don't end up having to turn to unhealthy alternatives. While this might seem like common sense, it will likely take some preparation to ensure you are ready to go when the time is right. While this means the overall time commitment required for the diet is likely steeper than others, once you get into the habit of preparing your food all at once you may find it actually saves you time in the long run. What's more, it will ensure that you are always able to choose the keto option, removing choice from the equation completely. it will also make it easier to eat smaller portions, decrease your salt intake and more easily track the specifics, including calories, when compared with rolling the dice on meals out.

Stay on track: In order to ensure you are on the right track, you are going to want to test yourself while you are in the transition phase. There are many different tests for ketosis, including blood tests and urine strips. What is being tested for in these instances is a substance known as acetone which is created when a ketone is broken down into energy. Overall, you are going to be looking for a ketone level of 3, as this will show your body is properly in ketosis. If you go over this number, you are going to want to increase the number of calories you eat per day as it is a sign that your body isn't getting enough essential nutrients. Finally, once you are in ketosis you can monitor your day to day progress by being aware of a metallic taste on your tongue and a slightly overripe apple smell on your breath.

When it comes to cutting out your carbohydrates, some people's bodies need a little more help making it into ketosis. If testing reveals that you are having a difficult time inching past the .5 mark, then you may need to reconsider the amount of protein that is still a part of your diet. If you consume an excess of protein then it becomes glucose, which raises your insulin levels just like glucose created from carbs. If you can't seem to cut out the extra protein, add in more fat to balance things out. Start by adding a tablespoon of coconut oil and a tablespoon of melted butter to your morning coffee or tee and go from there. Not only will this help you to feel fuller in the mornings, it will make you less likely to seek out unhealthy carbs instead.

Avoid grazing: While fully transitioning into the keto diet will help to ensure that you feel less full, overall, this change won't happen overnight. Until you find the right mix of macronutrients for your body, you may find yourself regularly feeling hungrier than before. While this is the case, it is important to make a conscious effort to eat full meals, as opposed to grazing on snacks, even keto approved snacks as this is a great way to stall the initial onslaught of weight loss that typically comes with the ketogenic transition. While a fat bomb or two per day is fine, they can add up quickly if you aren't paying attention, depriving you of the results of all of your hard work in the process.

Eat natural: When it comes to refilling your pantry with keto-approved items, it is important to stick with all-natural items in addition to those that are simply low in carbohydrates as the more processed an item is the less room that is going to be left for nutritional value. However, it is not enough to simply look for items that are marked as low-carb, as this has become a marking phrase in line with no sugar added and fat free which may more may not have any actual bearing on the nutritional content of the item in question.

On the contrary, items that are truly healthy don't need to advertise this fact, the fat to carb ratio of an avocado isn't subject to debate which means you never have to worry if it is actually as healthy as the label says. Avoid hype when it comes to what you put into your body, seek out organic, natural foods as much as possible.

Chapter 2

Keto Kitchen essentials for meal preparation

All these are the Basics you will want to get fast and simple keto-friendly foods. If you do not already have them, then it is simple to buy from somewhere.

Skillet

For the maximum for your buck, put money into a cast iron skillet that can continue to cooking for several decades. All these are simple to wash and safer than having a cheap Teflon-covered pan -- also it will help to keep your iron levels up.

Knives

Very Excellent knives are Necessary for any meal preparation. High quality is critical here, as low-quality knives may slide and slide, which makes them a possible hazard. Start looking for a suitable chef's knife which will enable you to cut and slice easily.

Slow cooker

There is a slow cooker Fantastic for "forgetting and setting" your keto foods since they cook. It's simple to throw everything and let it work its magic as you do anything else. An Immediate Pot is a beneficial tool for rapidly making homemade both meats and sauces.

Parchment papers

Parchment paper is perfect for preventing sticking after baking soda, whether it's at a casserole dish or onto a baking sheet.

Glass food container

If you operate away From the house, containers allow you to break recipes up to individual servings to catch and move. Glass is far much better than vinyl since it is dishwasher safe, and retains the damaging compounds in plastic from the entire human physique.

While these choices are not necessities for supper snacking, they could make the process simpler (and far more pleasurable).

Blender

Blenders are cheap, not as bulky and ideal for beating eggs, mixing noodles, which makes sauces such as mayo and whipping cream and much more.

Vegetable Spiralizer

A ton of cash if you adore fermented "pasta," such as zucchini noodles. As you are able to purchase pre-spiralizer veggies in the shop, it is cheaper to create your own in your home.

If you intend to consider your meals, you require a kitchen scale. This can be helpful for those brand fresh the keto diet who are trying hard to remain in ketosis and wish to be precise.

Chapter 3

Keto breakfast choices

Baked bacon omelet

Total Prep & Cooking Time: 25 min.

Yields: 2 Servings

Ingredients

- 4 eggs
- 142g. bacon cut in cubes
- 85g. butter
- 56g. fresh spinach
- 15g.minced chives
- Table salt and pepper

Instructions

1. Grease an individual dish with butter.
2. Fry bacon and spinach in the butter.

3. Whisk the eggs mix in the spinach and bacon, including the fat made from skillet.

4. Add some chopped chives. Season to taste with pepper and salt.

5. Dispense the egg combination to a baking dish and bake for twenty minutes until set and golden brown.

6. Let cool for a couple of minutes and function. Nutrition Facts: Calories: 737kcl | Protein: 21 g | Net Carbs: 2 g | Fat: 72g|

Spring veggie and goat cheese omelet

Total Prep & Cooking Time: 25min.

Yields: 2 Servings

Ingredients

- 4 eggs
- 30ml heavy whipping cream
- 15g. butter
- 4 asparagus, chopped into pieces
- salt and pepper

- 1 cup of baby spinach

- 56g. goat cheese

- 0.5 scallion, sliced

Instructions

1. Twist together the eggs and the cream until well blended. Put aside.

2. Heat the butter a sizable skillet over moderate heat till melted. Remove to a bowl or a bowl, then maintaining the peanut butter from the pan.

3. Reduce heat to Low and allow the pan cool a couple of minutes, then pour into the egg mix. Let cook undisturbed till the borders have been set, then raise the edges lightly with a spatula and allow the eggs in the middle run under to cook.

4. When the center is mostly put, sprinkle with pepper and salt. Then organize the egg and cooked asparagus within half of that available omelet. Crumble the goat cheese with your palms.

5. Flip another half of this omelet over and cook an additional minute or 2. With green onion. Nutrition Facts: Calories: 339kcl | Protein: 19 g | Net Carbs: 2 g | Fat: 28g|

Bacon cheddar cornbread waffles with egg and bacon

Total Prep & Cooking Time: 20min.

Yields: 2 Servings

Ingredients

- 15g. coconut flour
- 0.1 cup oat fiber
- 0.1 cup unflavored whey protein isolate
- 0.4 tsp baking powder
- 0.1 tsp salt
- 28g.melted butter
- 0.1 cup coconut oil, melted
- 15ml water
- 1 egg
- 0.25 tsp corn extract (optional)
- 60g cheddar cheese

- 0.5scallion, chopped
- 28g. cooked bacon, chopped

Instructions:

1. Prepare waffle iron as manufacturer directs.

2. Combine all ingredients. Add water, coconut oil, eggs, and the butter. Stir in the corn extract, cheese, cheese, scallions, and celery.

3. Scoop the mixture into the waffle iron Careful not to overfill the wells. Cook till and is browned slightly crisp. Serve warm.

Nutrition Facts: Calories: 327kcl | Protein: 11 g | Net Carbs: 1 g | Fat: 31g|

Avocado eggs and bacon sails

Total Prep & Cooking Time: 20min.

Yields: 2 Servings

Ingredients

- 1 boiled egg
- 0.25 avocado
- 0.5 tsp olive oil
- 5g. bacon

- Pepper and salt

Instructions:

1. Place the eggs in a sauce skillet and spread with water. Bring to a light bubble and let stew for 8-10 minutes. Spot the eggs in super cold water promptly when they are done to make them simpler to strip.
2. Cut the eggs into equal parts the long way and scoop out the yolks. Spot them in a little bowl.
3. Add oil and avocado and mash until blended, add salt and pepper taste.
4. It takes approximately 5--7 minutes. You might also fry them.
5. With a spoon, carefully insert the mixture into the egg that is cooked Whites and place the bacon! Enjoy!
   Nutrition Facts: Calories: 144kcl | Protein: 5g | Net Carbs: 1 g | Fat: 13g|

Frittata with fresh spinach

Total Prep & Cooking Time: 25min.

Yields: 2 Servings

Ingredients

- 79g. diced bacon
- 15g, butter
- 113g. fresh spinach
- 4 eggs
- 0.5cup heavy whipping cream
- 70g. cheese, grated
- Pepper and salt

Instructions:

1. Turn on the oven to 175c and Grease a baking dish
2. Fry the bacon in butter on medium heat. Insert the spinach and stir fry until wilted. Remove the pan from the heat.
3. Whisk the eggs and cream and pour it into a baking dish.

4. Add spinach, the bacon, and cheese on upper and spot in the middle of the oven. cook for 25-- 30 minutes or until brown.

   Nutrition Facts: Calories: 661kcl | Protein: 27g | Net Carbs: 4 g | Fat: 59g|

Salad sandwiches

Total Prep & Cooking Time:10 min.

Yields: 2 Servings

Ingredients

- 0.25cups Romaine lettuce or baby gem lettuce
- 0.5oz. butter
- O.5 cups of cheese of your liking
- 0.5 Avocado
- One cherry tomatoes

Instructions

1. Rinse the lettuce thoroughly and then apply as a foundation for those toppings.

2. Smear butter on the lettuce leaves, slit the cheese, tomato, and avocado and put in on top. Nutrition Facts: Calories: 374kcl | Protein: 10g | Net Carbs: 3g | Fat: 34g|

Garlic bread

Total Prep & Cooking Time: 30min.

Yields: 2 Servings

Ingredients

Garlic butter

- Garlic butter
- 1/4cup. butter, at room temperature
- 0.25 garlic clove, minced

- 0.5 tbsp. finely chopped, parsley

- 0.125tsp salt

- Bread

- 63g. almond flour

- 16g. ground psyllium husk powder

- 2.5g baking powder

- 0.25tsp sea salt

- 0.5tsp cider vinegar or white wine vinegar

- 0.25cup boiling water

- 0.75 egg white

Instructions

1. Preheat the oven 175c
2. Boil and include the vinegar and egg whites into the bowl, even while stirring using a hand mixer for approximately 30 minutes. Do not overmix the dough the consequences should resemble Play-Doh.
3. Type with hands To 10 pieces and roll up to hot dog buns. Be certain that you leave enough distance between them to the baking sheet to double in size.

4. Bake on in the oven for 40-50 minutes; then they are done once you're able to hear a hissing noise when tapping on the base of the bun.

5. Create the butter Mix together and place it in the refrigerator.

6. Take out the buns of the oven when they are done and depart to allow cool. Just take the butter from the refrigerator. If the buns are chilled, cut them in halves, then with a serrated knife and distribute garlic butter on each half.

7. Turn up your oven to 425°F (225°C) and inhale the garlic for 10-15 minutes, till golden brown. Nutrition Facts: Calories: 92kcl | Protein: 2g | Net Carbs: 1g | Fat: 9g|

Tuna salad with capers

Total Prep & Cooking Time: 15min.

Yields: 2 Servings

Ingredients

- 56g. tuna in olive oil

- 51g mayonnaise

- 12g cream fraiche

- 0.5 tbsp. capers

- 0.25 finely chopped leek

- 0.25tsp chili flakes

- salt and pepper

Instructions

1. Drain the tuna
2. Mix all the ingredients, season with salt and chili or pepper flakes. You are all set!
3. Serve with eggs.

Nutrition Facts: Calories: 271kcl | Protein: 89g | Net Carbs: 1g | Fat: 26g|

Cheese roll-ups

Total Prep & Cooking Time: min.

Yields: 2 Servings

Ingredients

- ½ cup cheddar cheese, in slices

- 0.02 cup butter

Instructions

1. Set the cheese slices.

2. Slice butter or trim on bits that are thin with a knife.

3. Cover with the rolls and then butter up. Serve as a snack.

Nutrition Facts: Calories: 335kcl | Protein: 13g | Net Carbs: 2g | Fat: 31g|

Salami and Brie cheese plate

Total Prep & Cooking Time: 10min.

Yields: 2 Servings

Ingredients

- 1 cup Brie cheese
- ½ cup salami
- 1/4 lettuce
- 1 avocado
- 0.5 cup macadamia nuts
- 0.25 cup olive oil

Instructions

1. Put avocado, salami, lettuce, cheese and nuts. Drizzle oil on the salad and serve.

Nutrition Facts: Calories: 1203kcl | Protein: 21g | Net Carbs: 3g | Fat: 34g.

Breakfast tapas

Total Prep & Cooking Time: 15min.

Yields: 2 Servings

Ingredients

- Cheese mozzarella, or cheddar.
- Cold cuts salami, ham, chorizo, and prosciutto.
- Pickled cucumbers, peppers, radishes, Cucumber.
- Mayonnaise with pepper and avocado.
- Nuts(hazelnuts, almonds or walnuts)
- Basil

Instructions

1. Cut the vegetables and chees into cubes or sticks.
2. Divide the avocado and cut into pieces.
3. 1 tsp of crushed peppercorns mix with 1 cup of mayonnaise and add freshly squeezed lemon juice.
4. Serve in the avocado shells.
   Nutrition Facts: Calories: 527kcl | Protein: 18g | Net Carbs: 4g | Fat: 45g.

Low-carb tortillas

Total Prep & Cooking Time: min.

Yields: 2 Servings

Ingredients

- 0.75 egg
- 0.75 egg white
- 42g. cream cheese
- 0.5 tsp ground psyllium husk powder
- 0.3 tbsp. coconut flour
- 0.25 tsp salt

Instructions

1. Turn on the stove to 400°F

2. Beat an egg. Proceed to beat for a couple of minutes.

3. In a little bowl, then add coconut milk, salt, and psyllium. Add the flour mixture and blend well. Allow the batter sit for a couple of minutes, till it becomes thick, such as pancake batter. The batter stinks based upon the new psyllium husk powder.

4. Bring two sheets of parchment paper onto each. With a spatula, spread the batter (no longer than 1/4 inch thick) to 4--6 bands or two rectangles.

5. Bake for approximately 5 minutes or longer on the rack, till it turns brown.

6. Serve with your choice. We adore them together with salsa and ground beef! Also, cheese is a winner.

Nutrition Facts: Calories: 116kcl | Protein: 5g | Net Carbs: 2g | Fat: 70g.

Poppy-seed bread

Total Prep & Cooking Time: 30min.

Yields: 2 Servings

Ingredients

- Leafy greens
- Cherry tomatoes
- Mayonnaise, flavored with curry
- Cooked turkey or chicken
- 1/4. Cottage cheese
- 0.75egg
- 0.25 tbsp. olive oil
- 1tbs flaxseed or chia seed
- 1tbs sunflower seeds
- 0.25tsp baking powder
- 0.25tsp psyllium husk powder
- 0.25tsp sea salt
- 0.25tbsp poppy seeds

Instructions

1. Place all the dry ingredients. Mix it in oil, egg and cottage cheese. Sit for 15 minutes.
2. Evenly spread the batter on a parchment paper. Bake it for 25 minutes at 350°F (175°C).
3. Without the parchment paper, let it dry.
4. Cut into pieces and enjoy with toppings and butter.
5. You can serve the bread with a salad, a filling curry chicken mayonnaise.

Nutrition Facts: Calories: 128kcl | Protein: 7g | Net Carbs: 2g | Fat: 9g

Banana waffles

Total Prep & Cooking Time: 25 min.

Yields: 2 Servings

Ingredients

- 0.25 ripe banana
- One egg

- 38g almond flour
- 45ml coconut milk
- 0.25tbsp ground psyllium husk powder
- 0.25 pinch salt
- 0.25tsp baking powder
- 0.25tsp vanilla extract
- 0.25 tsp ground cinnamon
- Butter or coconut oil, for frying

Instructions

1. Mix all of the ingredients and let it sit for a few minutes
2. Fry in a frying pan with coconut oil or make in a waffle maker butter.
3. Serve with hazelnut spread or whipped coconut cream.
4. You can serve with fresh berries, or have them as is with melted butter.
   Nutrition Facts: Calories: 155kcl | Protein: 5g | Net Carbs: 4g | Fat: 13g.

Deviled eggs

Total Prep & Cooking Time: 15min.

Yields: 2 Servings

Ingredients

- 2 eggs
- 0.5 tsp Tabasco
- 1 oz. mayonnaise
- 0.5 pinch salt
- 4 strips of cooked smoked salmon or peeled shrimp
- Fresh Dill.

Instructions

1. boil the eggs by placing them in a pot
2. Boil for 8-10 minutes to make sure the eggs are hardboiled.
3. Eliminate the eggs from the pot and place in an ice bath for a few minutes
4. Cut half and scoop out the yolks.
5. Place the egg whites on a plate.

6. Mash the egg yolks and add mayonnaise, tobacco, and salt

7. Add the mixture to the egg whites and top with a shrimp on a piece of smoked salmon.

8. Decorate with dill.

   Nutrition Facts: Calories: 163kcl | Protein: 7g | Net Carbs: 0.5g | Fat: 15g.

Chapter 4

Lunchtime Dishes

Pimiento cheese meatballs

Total Prep & Cooking Time: 20 min.

Yields: 2 Servings

Ingredients

- Pimiento cheese
- 1oz mayonnaise
- 15g pickled jalapeños or pimientos
- 0.5 tsp chili powder or paprika powder
- 0.5 tbsp Dijon mustard
- 0.5 pinch cayenne pepper
- 0.25cup cheddar cheese grated

Meatballs

- 2 cup. ground beef
- Half an egg
- Pepper and salt

- 15g butter, for frying

Instructions

1. Mix all the ingredients for the pimiento cheese in a bowl. Leave it for 5 minutes.
2. Add egg and beef to the mixture and mix evenly. Add pepper and salt to taste.
3. Make meatballs and fry them in butter in a skillet on medium heat until they are properly cooked.
4. Serve with a side dish (mayonnaise or a salad) Nutrition Facts: Calories: 660kcl | Protein: 42g | Net Carbs: 1g | Fat: 53g

Chicken and cabbage plate

Total Prep & Cooking Time: 20 min.

Yields: 2 Servings

Ingredients

- 450g rotisserie chickens
- 200g. fresh green cabbage
- 0.5 red onion
- 15ml olive oil

- 0.5 cup mayonnaise
- Pepper and salt

Instructions

1. Cut the cabbage using a sharp knife place on a plate.
2. Slice the onion evenly and thinly. Place it on the plate, together with the mayonnaise and rotisserie chicken.
3. Add olive oil over the cabbage and some salt and pepper to taste.
   Nutrition Facts: Calories: 1041kcl | Protein: 48g | Net Carbs: 4g | Fat: 91g.

Roast beef and cheddar plate

Total Prep & Cooking Time: 15min.

Yields: 2 Servings

Ingredients

- 1cup. deli roast beef
- 3/4. cheddar cheese
- 1 avocado
- 6 radishes
- 1 scallion
- 0.5 cup mayonnaise
- 15g Dijon mustard
- 1/4cup. lettuce
- 30ml olive oil
- Pepper and salt

Instructions

1. Place avocado, cheese, radishes, and roast beef on a plate.
2. Add mayonnaise, mustard, and sliced onion.
3. Serve with olive oil and lettuce.
   Nutrition Facts: Calories: 1072kcl | Protein: 38g | Net Carbs: 5g | Fat: 95g.

Pork scaloppini

Total Prep & Cooking Time: 25min.

Yields: 2 Servings

Ingredients

- 0.75 lb boneless, thin cut pork chops
- ground black pepper and salt
- 0.5tbsp olive oil
- 1.5 tbsp. butter
- 15g capers
- 0.5cup chicken broth
- 15ml lemon juice
- 10 cherry tomatoes
- 15 g chopped parsley

Instructions

1. Season the pork chops evenly with pepper and salt
2. Heat the olive in a pan over moderate heat. Keep pork in the pan and cook until browned, 2 minutes for each side. Expel from the container and spread to keep warm.

3. Add the butter and the capers to the same pan and Cook until the capers are hot.

4. Using a rubber spatula include the lemon juice and chicken soup to the skillet. Mix it thoroughly.

5. Rise the temperature and boil until the sauce has reduced by about half.

6. Decrease the warmth and add the tomatoes to the container. Cook until slightly blistered and soft about 3 minutes.

7. Place the pork on a plate and pour the sauce over the top. Garnish with fresh parsley

Nutrition Facts: Calories: 461kcl | Protein: 35g | Net Carbs: 3g | Fat: 33g.

Caprese chicken

Total Prep & Cooking Time: 30min.

Yields: 2 Servings

Ingredients

- 0.75lb chicken breasts
- 15ml olive oil

- 0.5tsp sea salt
- 0.5 tsp Italian seasoning
- 0.25 tsp garlic powder
- 0.25 tsp ground black pepper
- 1/2cup. fresh mozzarella cheese, sliced
- 1 sliced tomato
- 30g basil, cut into long, thin strips
- 15ml balsamic vinegar
-

Instructions

1. heat the oven to 375°f
2. Spray the olive oil over the chicken breasts. Season with Italian seasoning in a bowl and Refrigerate for 20 minutes.
3. Heat skillet over medium-high heat. Fry the chicken breasts about 3 minutes.
4. Place the skillet to the oven and bake for 20 minutes.
5. Remove the skillet from the oven and spread the top of chicken breast with tomatoes and mozzarella. Bake in the oven for 3 minutes.
6. Drizzle the top of the chicken breast with vinegar and basil before serving.

Nutrition Facts: Calories: 553kcl | Protein: 50g | Net Carbs: 4g | Fat: 36g.

Lamb stew with dill sauce and green beans

Total Prep & Cooking Time: 35min.

Yields: 2 Servings

Ingredients

- 300g lamb, cut in bite-sized pieces
- water
- 0.5tsp white peppercorns,
- 0.5bay leaf
- ⅓ cup yellow onion
- 0.5carrot, sliced into circles
- 0.5 tbsp. salt
- 0.4cup heavy whipping cream
- 0.5tsp vinegar
- 0.2 finely chopped fresh dill
- 0.4lb fresh green beans
-

Instructions

1. Cut the meat into pieces. Place meat in the pot filled with water. Boil properly for a few minutes, then rinse meat to avoid having to skim the foam.
2. Place meat in the pot. Add dill, onion and carrot slices. Fill the water to cover and add salt and boil.
3. Remove broth and meat. Place the vegetables aside.
4. Pour the same amount of broth and cream in the pot. Boil and simmer for 15 minutes. Add salt, pepper, and vinegar
5. Place meat in the pot and warm and add chopped dill.
6. Boil green beans for 3-4 minutes. Serve together.

Nutrition Facts: Calories: 590kcl | Protein: 29g | Net Carbs: 4g | Fat: 49g.

Oven-baked Brie cheese

Total Prep & Cooking Time: 35min.

Yields: 2 Servings

Ingredients

- ½ cup. Brie cheese
- 0.2 cup. Walnuts or pecan
- 0.5 garlic clove
- 0.5tbsp fresh rosemary
- 0.5tbsp olive oil
- Pepper and salt
-

Instructions

1. Heat the oven to 400°F.Place the cheese on a sheet pan with parchment paper.
2. Chop the nuts and herbs and mince garlic. With the olive oil mix all. Add pepper and salt.
3. Place the chopped nut on the cheese and bake for 10 minutes.
4. Servc.

Nutrition Facts: Calories: 344kcl | Protein: 14g | Net Carbs: 1g | Fat: 31g.

Cauliflower hash browns

Total Prep & Cooking Time: 25min.

Yields: 2 Servings

Ingredients

- 0.5lb cauliflower
- 2 eggs
- 0.25   chopped onion
- 0.5tsp salt
- 1 pinch pepper
- 56g. butter, for frying

Instructions

1. grill the cauliflower using a food processor
2. Add remaining ingredients and cauliflower in a bowl and mix. Leave for 10 minutes.

3. Melt the butter in moderate heat in a skillet.

4. Place the grated cauliflower mixture in the skillet and level them evenly until they measure about 5 inches in diameter.

5. Fry for 5 minutes on each side.

Nutrition Facts: Calories: 342kcl | Protein: 31g | Net Carbs: 5g | Fat: 21g.

BBQ chicken with bacon

Total Prep & Cooking Time: 25min.

Yields: 2 Servings

Ingredients

Meatza crust

- 0.5 lb ground chicken
- 0.25tsp salt
- 1 cup powdered parmesan cheese

BBQ sauce

- 0.25 cup tomato sauce
- 0.5tsp cider vinegar
- 0.25tsp liquid smoke
- 0.25 tsp onion powder

- 0.25tsp garlic powder
- 00.25 tsp salt

Toppings

- 0.5 cup shredded cheese
- 0.25 onion
- 85g. bacon

Instructions

1. heat the oven to 425°
2. Ground chicken, parmesan, and salt mix thoroughly in a bowel.
3. Apply Grease on the parchment paper and add the crust mixture on the parchment and flatten evenly until it form 25cm in diameter.
4. Slide the crust with a piece of parchment paper onto the baking sheet.
5. Until the crust is turning brown, bake for 12 to 15 minutes

Nutrition Facts: Calories: 342kcl | Protein: 31g | Net Carbs: 5g | Fat: 21g.

Keto meatballs with mozzarella cheese

Total Prep & Cooking Time: 30min.

Yields: 2 Servings

Ingredients

- 0.5lb ground beef
- 35g. parmesan cheese, grated
- 0.5egg
- 0.25 tbsp. basil, dried
- 0.25tsp powdered onion
- 0.5 tsp powder garlic
- 0.5 tsp salt
- 0.25 tsp black pepper, grounded
- 1.25 tbsp. olive oil
- 200g. tomatoes, canned
- 1 tbsp. fresh parsley, finely chopped
- 100g. fresh spinach
- 30g. butter
- 75tg. fresh mozzarella cheese
- salt and pepper

Instructions

1. Blend thoroughly, egg, ground beef, parmesan cheese, salt and spices in a bowl.
2. make the balls about 30g of each from the mixture
3. Fry the meatballs until their golden brown on all sides with the olive oil in a skillet.
4. Put cooker to moderate heat and add the canned tomatoes, while stirring simmer it for 15 minutes.
5. Season with pepper and salt to taste. Stir it after adding the parsley.
6. fry the spinach for few minutes with the butter in a separate pan
7. With mozzarella cheese on top add the spinach to the meatball. Divided into pieces and Serve.

Nutrition Facts: Calories: 622kcl | Protein: 39g | Net Carbs: 4g | Fat: 49g.

Naan bread with melted garlic butter

Total Prep & Cooking Time: 30min.

Yields: 2 Servings

Garlic butter

Ingredient

- 113g. butter
- 2 garlic cloves,
- 0.75 cup coconut flour
- 30g psyllium husk powder
- 2.5g onion, powdered
- 0.5 tsp baking powder
- 5g salt
- 0.25 cup coconut oil
- 500ml boiling water
- salt

1. Combination all waterless components in a bowl and make a doh.
2. .It should resemble the consistency of Play-Doh

3. Cut into pieces and make balls and evenly spread with your hands on parchment paper.

4. Fry the Naan on skillet until turn a nice brown color.

5. Add the garlic to melted butter and Apply it on the bread

6. Add salt according to your taste.

Nutrition Facts: Calories: 601kcl | Protein: 30g | Net Carbs: 5g | Fat: 43g.

Butter-fried kale with pork and cranberries

Total Prep & Cooking Time: 30min.

Yields: 2 Servings

Ingredients

- 1.5oz. butter
- 0.5lb kale
- 170g bacon
- 30g. pecans or walnuts
- 0.5 cup frozen cranberries
- salt black pepper

Instructions.

1. Wash and cut kale into large chunks.
2. Fry the bacon in butter over moderate heat until brown and crispy.
3. Place kale in the pan and fry fora few minutes until wilted. Add Salt and pepper.
4. Place cranberries and nuts in the pan and stir and serve it.

Nutrition Facts: Calories: 749kcl | Protein: 14g | Net Carbs: 8g | Fat: 73g.

Butter fried fish with tandoori sauce

Total Prep & Cooking Time: 30min.

Yields: 2 Servings

Ingredients

- 1.5cups sour cream
- 6tsp tandoori seasoning
- 450g cauliflower

- 30ml olive oil
- 1.5lbs any white fish with skin
- 60g. butter
- salt and pepper

Instructions

1. heat the stove to 430°F
2. Tandoori seasoning with sour cream. Add Salt and pepper to taste.
3. Cut the cauliflower into tiny sections and place in a preparing dish and sprinkle with olive oil. Bake until it gets a beautiful brown color.
4. Add Salt and pepper on the two sides of fish. Sear skin side down in butter on moderate warmth. Broil until the skin gets firm and the meat cooks appropriately.
5. Serve fish with cauliflower and tandoori sauce.

Nutrition Facts: Calories: 592kcl | Protein: 35g | Net Carbs: 3g | Fat: 38g.

Creamed green cabbage with chorizo

Total Prep & Cooking Time: 30min.

Yields: 2 Servings

Ingredients

- 700g. green cabbage
- 60g. butter
- 1.25cups whipping cream
- Pepper and salt
- 125g parsley, chopped
- 0.5 lemon,
-

Fried chorizo

- 700g. chorizo
- 30g butter

Instructions

1. Fry the chorizo with the butter moderate heat.

2. Place cabbage in the butter on moderate heat and Stir it until cabbage is nice brown color

3. Add whipping cream, and boil it. Turn off the heat, and let simmer it. Add pepper and salt to taste

4. Before serving with the fried chorizo, add lemon and parsley.

   Nutrition Facts: Calories: 1260kcl | Protein: 47g | Net Carbs: 7g | Fat: 112g.

Buttery harissa shrimp skewers

Total Prep & Cooking Time: 20min.

Yields: 2 Servings

Ingredients

- 0.5 lb large shrimp, peeled and deveined
- ground pepper and salt
- 1.5tbsp butter, melted
- 3 tsp harissa paste

- 0.5tbsp fresh lime juice
- 0.25sea salt
- 1 garlic clove
- 0.5 a lime
- two (10-inch) skewers

Instructions

1. Season the shrimp evenly with pepper and salt.
2. Place the, harissa, lime juice, butter, garlic, and salt in a bowl.
3. Place the shrimp in the vessel and cover it in the sauce. Leave it for 1 hour.
4. Pour any remaining marinade over top, After the Threading the shrimp onto the skewers.
5. Heat a grill pan and place the skewers in the pan and cook properly
6. With the lime wedges, serve it.

Nutrition Facts: Calories: 1260kcl | Protein: 47g | Net Carbs: 7g | Fat: 112g.

Chapter 5

Dinner specialities

Oven-baked chicken in garlic butter

Total Prep & Cooking Time: 60 min.

Yields: 2 Servings

Ingredients

- 1.5lbs chicken breast
- 1/3 tabs salt
- 0.25tsp black pepper powder
- 60g. butter
- One garlic

Instructions

1. Heat the oven to 400°F and mix the chicken with pepper and salt.
2. Place chicken breast in prepared baking dish.
3. Mix the butter and garlic in a pan over moderate heat for to melt the butter.

4. Leave the butter to reduce the heat for a few minutes.

5. Apply the butter garlic mixture inside and over the chicken. Bake it on down oven rack 1 hour.

6. Take away the extracts from the lowest part of the pan every 1/3 hours.

7. Serve it with the juice as a side dish of your choice.

Nutrition Facts: Calories: 996kcl | Protein: 59g | Net Carbs: 1g | Fat: 83g.

Sandwich with smoked salmon and horseradish cream

Total Prep & Cooking Time: 15 min.

Yields: 2 Servings

Ingredients

- 200g. smoked salmon
- 0.5cup sour cream or mayonnaise
- 30g. grated fresh horseradish

Mug bread

- 30g almond flour
- 30g coconut flour

- 1.5tsp baking powder
- 0.25 tsp salt
- Two eggs
- 30g whipping cream
- 5g butter

For Serving

- 30g butter
- 0.5oz. arugula lettuce
- 0.25 finely sliced zucchini, (optional)

Instructions

1. Cut the salmon into pieces and mix with grated horseradish and mayonnaise. Leave it in the refrigerator until served.
2. For the bread, Mix all dry ingredients. mix the cracked egg with the cream. Beat until it gets smooth. Pour into greased glass molds.
3. Microwave the bread for 2 minutes (700 watts).
4. Leave to reduce heat and remove from the mug. Cut it into pieces.
5. Spread butter on each slice, add sliced zucchini, lettuce leaves, horseradish cream and a dollop of the salmon on to butter shredded slices.

Nutrition Facts: Calories: 1025kcl | Protein: 70g | Net Carbs: 4g | Fat: 80g.

Zucchini salmon fritters

Total Prep & Cooking Time: 30 min.

Yields: 2 Servings

Ingredients

For the homemade tartar sauce:

- 0.5tbsp mayonnaise
- 0.5tbsp Greek yogurt
- 0.25tbsp whipping cream, heavy
- 5g fresh horseradish
- 0.5dill pickle
- 0.5tbsp scallions
- 0.25 tbsp fresh dill
- 5ml apple cider vinegar
- pepper and salt

Zucchini salmon fritters

- 200g salmon canned
- 0.5   grated zucchini
- 5g chopped onions
- 0.5 tbsp. psyllium husk powder
- 0.5 egg
- 0.5 tsp salt
- 0.25tsp pepper
- 70g. butter

Instructions

1. Mix grated zucchini, onion, salmon, psyllium, egg, salt, and pepper in a mixing bowl. Stir appropriately with a spatula until all ingredients are evenly mixed. Leave aside for a few minutes.
2. Cut dill, scallion, and pickle and in a bowl and add to yogurt, whipping cream, horseradish, and mayonnaise. Add salt, pepper, and vinegar.
3. On moderate heat, heat the frying pan and Melt the butter. Using spatula add finely mix fritter mixture into the pan.
4. Harden the fritter mixture flat using spatula. And make it nice round fritters. Cook properly until golden on one side, then flip.
5. Serve with a side salad and tartar sauce.

Nutrition Facts: Calories: 523kcl | Protein: 25g | Net Carbs: 3g | Fat: 45g.

Beetroot-cured salmon with dill oil

Total Prep & Cooking Time: 60 min.

Yields: 2 Servings

Ingredients

- 0.5 beet
- 15g salt
  0.25peppercorns
- 0.5 lime
- 0.5 lb salmon

Dill oil

- 0.25 cup chopped fresh dill
- 0.25tbsp spinach, frozen
- 0.25 cup light olive oil
- pepper and salt

Serving

- 30g. sliced daikon

- 0.25 lb lettuce

Instructions

1. Rinse and peel the beetroot. Grate and place in a bowl. Add salt and lime add white peppercorn.
2. Apply the flesh side properly with the beetroot mixture. While placing the salmon skin side down.
3. Place the salmon in a crystal bowl and shield it. Leave it in the refrigerator for 60 minutes.
4. Mix spinach and dill in a blender. Add pepper, salt and olive oil to taste.
5. Open the salmon and wash off the beetroot cure.
6. Divide the fish into slices. Serve with lettuce, daikon, and dill oil.
   Nutrition Facts: Calories: 500kcl | Protein: 20g | Net Carbs: 3g | Fat: 77g.

Sashimi rolls

Total Prep & Cooking Time: 60 min.

Yields: 2 Servings

Ingredients

- 200g. salmon or fresh tuna
- five nori sheets
- 0.25cup soy sauce
- 30mlolive oil
- 1/3bs sesame seeds
- One lime

Instructions

1. cut the fish in to long pieces
2. With water, apply the nori sheets. Place them flat on a wooden surface and roll a fish pieces one by one. Leave it for few minutes.
3. Crosswise, cut the rolls into small pieces.
4. Mix the olive oil, sesame seeds and soy sauce in a separate bowl.
5. With the sauce and lime wedges, Serve the sashimi.

   Nutrition Facts: Calories: 372kcl | Protein: 21g | Net Carbs: 5g | Fat: 68g.

Ham & cheese quiche with cauliflower crust

Total Prep & Cooking Time: 30 min.

Yields: 2 Servings

Ingredients

Crust

- 120g. cauliflower florets, riced
- 5g grated parmesan cheese
- 0.5 egg
- 0.25tsp salt
- 0.25 tsp black pepper

Filling

1. 60g. smoked deli ham, cubed or diced
2. 40g. shredded cheddar cheese
3. 1.5eggs
4. 0.25cup whipping cream
5. 0.5 garlic clove, minced
6. pepper and salt

7.

Instructions

Crust

1. Place the cauliflower rice in a safe bowl and close it with plastic wrap. Until very soft, Cooke a few minutes. Drain the cauliflower through using the tea towel.
2. Transfer cauliflower into a bowl and heat the oven to 350°F.
3. Mix the egg, salt, pepper, and parmesan, until finely mixed. Apply butter on a ceramic plate and apply press to the cauliflower mixture until form flat evenly. Bake 15 minutes.

    Filling

4. Stove heat at 350°F and spread the cheese parmesan and ham over the cauliflower crust.
5. Beat the garlic eggs and cream until well mixed. Add salt and pepper to taste. Bake until properly cook quiche.

    Nutrition Facts: Calories: 281kcl | Protein: 30g | Net Carbs: 6g | Fat: 64g.

Salmon with pesto and spinach

Total Prep & Cooking Time: 25min.

Yields: 2 Servings

Ingredients

- 360g. salmon
- 0.5cup mayonnaise or sour cream
- 0.5 tbsp. green pesto or red pesto
- 0.5oz. grated parmesan cheese
- 0.05lb fresh spinach
- 0.5oz. butter
- salt and pepper

Instructions

1. Preheat the stove to 400°F
2. Apply butter on a baking dish. Pepper and salt place on the salmon fillets
3. Mix pesto, parmesan cheese, and mayonnaise, and apply over the salmon.
4. Bake the salmon until it properly cooks.
5. Fry the spinach in butter about 2 minutes. Season with pepper and salt.

6. Serve the meal with the salmon.

   Nutrition Facts: Calories: 902kcl | Protein: 20g | Net Carbs: 1g | Fat: 79g.

Cheese taco cups

Total Prep & Cooking Time: 20min.

Yields: 2 Servings

Cheese cups

- 16 pieces of preferred cheese
- Salsa
- Four diced tomatoes
- 90g onion
- One fresh diced jalapeno
- 15 ml of lime juice
- 90g cilantro

1. heat stove to 375
2. keep slices of cheese on a parchment sheet
3. Bake it for until starting to golden color at edges
4. Leave it for cool for a few minutes.

5. To form a cup shape, slowly place the slices in a muffin tin.

6. Leave it cool for a few minutes

Salsa

1. Place cilantro tomatoes, jalapeno, lime juice and onions in a covered bowl in the fridge for few minutes.

   Nutrition Facts: Calories: 300kcl | Protein: 18g | Net Carbs: 3g | Fat: 62g.

Broccoli cheese soup

Total Prep & Cooking Time: 20min.

Yields: 2 Servings

Ingredients

- 15gbutter
- 1 onion, chopped
- 2 garlic cloves,
- Pepper and salt
- 0.5tsb xanthan gum
- 0.5cup chicken broth

- One cup of broccoli
- One cup heavy cream
- 1.5 cups cheddar cheese

Instructions

1. Heat the pot on the oven. Place the garlic, salt, and pepper, and onions in the pot. Fry the onion until golden brown.
2. Add xanthan gum on the onions and butter. Mix in the chicken soup.
3. Position the broccoli in the pot. Confirm the vegetables are smeared with soup mixture.
4. Mix cream and xanthan gum quickly.
5. Carefully add cheese into the pot.
6. Add more broccoli and cheese on the top and serve

Nutrition Facts: Calories: 418kcl | Protein: 20g | Net Carbs: 5g | Fat: 32g.

Tex-Mex casserole

Total Prep & Cooking Time: 20min.

Yields: 2 Servings

Ingredients

- 0.75lb ground beef
- 30g.butter
- 0.5tbsp. Tex-Mex seasoning
- 1 oz. crushed tomatoes
- 30g. pickled jalapeños
- 1oz. shredded cheese

For serving

- 0.5 cup of sour cream
- 0.5 scallion
- 2.5oz leafy greens

Instructions

1. Heat the stove to 400°F.
2. On medium-high heat, fry the ground beef in butter until cooked properly.

3. Add crushed tomatoes and Tex-Mex seasoning.
   Mix and let simmer for a few minutes.

4. Grease the baking dish and Place the ground
   beef mixture on it. Place jalapeños and cheese on
   top of it.

5. Bake for 20 minutes

6. Mix sour cream with chopped scallion in a
   separate bowl.

7. Serve the casserole with a green salad.
   Nutrition Facts: Calories: 650kcl | Protein: 22g |
   Net Carbs: 6g | Fat: 69g.

Turkey plate

Total Prep & Cooking Time: 15min.

Yields: 2 Serving

Ingredients

- 180g. deli turkey
- Two avocados
- 90g. cream cheese
- 60g. lettuce

- 60ml olive oil
- Pepper and salt.

Instructions

1. Place the cheese, lettuce turkey, and sliced avocado on a plate.
2. Add olive oil over the vegetables and add pepper and salt.

Nutrition Facts: Calories: 450kcl | Protein: 35g | Net Carbs: 4g | Fat: 65g.

Cheese omelet

Total Prep & Cooking Time: 15min.

Yields: 2 Servings

Ingredients

- 90g. butter
- Six eggs
- 210g. cheddar cheese, shredded

- Salt and pepper

Instructions

1. Beat the eggs until smooth. Mix in 1/2 of the shredded cheddar. Add salt and pepper.
2. In a hot frying pan, melt the butter. put the egg blend and leave it for 5 minutes.
3. Reduce the heat and cook the egg mixture through. Add the left ½ of shredded cheese and serve.

Nutrition Facts: Calories: 500kcl | Protein: 60g | Net Carbs: 3g | Fat: 65g.

Fried halloumi cheese with mushrooms

Total Prep & Cooking Time: 18min.

Yields: 2 Servings

Ingredients

- 300g. mushrooms
- 300g. halloumi cheese
- 90g. butter
- Ten green olives

- salt and pepper
- 0.5cup mayonnaise

Instructions

1. Rinse and cut the mushrooms into slices.
2. In a frying pan, heat the butter.
3. Stir Fry the mushrooms on moderate heat for few minutes. Season with pepper and salt.
4. Serve with olives.
   Nutrition Facts: Calories: 600kcl | Protein: 55g | Net Carbs: 5g | Fat: 68g.

Goat cheese salad with balsamic butter

Total Prep & Cooking Time: 18min.

Yields: 2 Servings

Ingredients

- 300g. goat cheese
- 0.25cup pumpkin seeds

- 60g. butter

- 15ml balsamic vinegar

- 90g. baby spinach

Instructions

1. Turn on the stove to 400°F.

2. In a greased baking dish, Place the slices of goat cheese and bake for 10 minutes.

3. Fry the pumpkin seeds on a hot pan in a pan until they become a darker color.

4. Reduce the heat and add butter. Leave until it turns a brown color. Add vinegar and boil for a few more minutes.

5. Place the cheese on top of the flatten baby spinach plate. Add the balsamic butter.
   Nutrition Facts: Calories: 450kcl | Protein: 45g | Net Carbs: 6g | Fat: 60g.

Mackerel and egg plate

Total Prep & Cooking Time: 15min.

Yields: 2 Servings

Ingredients

- Four eggs
- 30g butter
- 1cup. canned mackerel in tomato sauce
- 60g. lettuce
- 0.5 red onion
- 0.25cup olive oil
- salt and pepper

Instructions

1. In butter, fry the eggs.
2. Add, thin slices of red onion, lettuce, and mackerel on a plate with the eggs. Spread the olive oil over the salad. Season to taste with salt and pepper.

Nutrition Facts: Calories: 560kcl | Protein: 55g | Net Carbs: 4g | Fat: 66g.

Chapter 6

7-day keto meal plan

This table is an example of a one-week meal plan to begin your journey with the right foot.

Days	Breakfast	lunch	Dinner
Monday	Cheese roll-ups	Pimiento cheese meatballs	Sashimi rolls
Tuesday	Tuna salad with capers	Chicken and cabbage plate	Zucchini salmon fritters

Wednesday	Breakfast tapas	Roast beef and cheddar plate	Sandwich with smoked salmon and horseradish cream
Thursday	Salad sandwiches	Pork scaloppini	Mackerel and egg plate
Friday	Salami and Brie cheese plate	Cauliflower hash browns	Goat cheese salad with balsamic butter
Saturday	Frittata with fresh spinach	Butter-fried kale with pork and cranberries	Fried halloumi cheese with mushrooms

Sunday	Avocado eggs and bacon sails	Butter fried fish with tandoori sauce	Cheese omelet

How to shed pounds rapid on a keto diet?

The famous formula for exercising more to eat less and lose weight is old, unreal, and unstable. What you eat, and Ketogenic Diet is a tool to lose weight where it is most prominent. Exercise promotes lean muscle building, greater bone electricity, and better stamina and balance. Exercise makes use of your glycogen keep, which enables you to get faster in the ketosis. Therefore, to reduce the weight, only to see these benefits, see exercise as a tool.

4 types of Exercises in Ketos

• Aerobic Exercise: Cardio Your heart rate lasts longer than three minutes. Low intensity, stable-state cardio is fat burning, so this keto is very suitable for the dieter.

• Anabolic exercise: HIIT or Weight education for muscle building. Intense, low bursts of strength to reinforce energy and speed. Carbohydrates are the primary gas for an anaerobic workout, so fat cannot provide enough power for this kind of workout.

• Exercise of Flexibility: Yoga and Stretch, to improve muscle and to speed up joints, and to prevent injuries due to lack of muscle over time.

• Stability practice: core training, Pilates, balance exercises, yoga Improve alignment, balance, muscular strength, and movement control.

When you are in Ketosis, the intensity of exercise is the best:

During low-depth cardio workout, the frame makes use of fats as its number one strength assets.

During excessive-depth aerobic exercising, carbohydrates are usually the primary strength assets.

This is the reason that when you calculate your macros, keep in mind your level of activity. When you start on a ketogenic diet, SKD (standard ketogenic diet) may not be enough to fuel your workout. Targeted Ketogenic Diet and Fat Adaptation
In TKD, you eat 15 to 30 grams fast-acting carbs within 30 minutes of your workout and 30 minutes after your workout. It provides glycogen in the proper amount of time to perform your muscles during training and to recover later.

The carbs you consume are used at once for this motive and save you the hazard of having out of the Ketosis. The property information is that for as long as you live in Ketosis, your body will become as fat-adaptive and is more efficient in burning fat for energy, a natural process that is lazy when your body is constantly supplied with carbs is done.

Alternating Fasting with the Keto Diet:

Intermittent fasting is frequently completed along with the ketogenic eating regimen. The two methods help every different. Fasting allows you get into Ketosis, and Ketosis facilitates you speedy greater effortlessly. Together, they burn loads of fat and can assist you to lose weight faster.

Benefits of Exercising in Ketosis

Far from obstructing exercises, Ketosis provides benefits to exercising, which increases its fitness to ordinary health and weight loss.

In one observe, compared to those who ate an excessive-carb diet, extremely-staying power athletes who ate a low-carb diet for as a minimum 20months, burnt 2-3 times more fat during the three-hour-long run. In the same study, we used a low-carb group and filled the same amount of muscle glycogen as a high-carb group. Being in Ketosis can help prevent fatigue during a long period of aerobic exercise. And Ketosis has been shown to help in the maintenance of blood glucose during exercise in obese individuals.

As mentioned above, the power of keto-optimization helps lower carb dieters perform better in all forms of exercise over time with reduced carbs.

Avoid overtraining. Overtraining increases the level of your cortisol. Cortisol, the stress hormone, your body thinks you are in battle or flight mode, increase your insulin and blood sugar, not you want on keto.

Nutritional Supplements on a Ketogenic Diet

•Electrolytes:

Adopting a ketogenic weight-reduction plan will exchange the manner your frame makes use of (and loses) certain minerals. Not replacing those minerals can cause signs and symptoms of the "keto flu" including light-headedness, headaches, constipation, muscle cramps, and fatigue. Refer to this text for tips on how to replace commonplace minerals which include sodium, potassium, magnesium, and calcium.

- Fish Oil

Fish oil is a fantastic supply of omega 3s and a natural anti-inflammatory. Consuming approximately 3000-5000 mg of fish oil according to today with excessive EPA/DHA is usually recommended. One first-rate source is Antarctic Krill Oil. Make sure that whichever supply you pick, it has the IFOS 5 famous person score and is stamped with a FOS approval.

- MCT Powder

MCT oil powder is a unique shape of dietary fat unexpectedly absorbed through the body and has a wide range of fitness advantages. Supplementation with MCT powder can help combat fatigue, suppress appetite, decorate thermogenesis, and assist your frame adapts to the usage of ketones for gasoline. A recent scientific assessment confirmed that MCTs should efficiently lower body weight, overall frame fats, hip circumference, waist circumference, general subcutaneous fat, and visceral fat.

- Collagen

Shown collagen is a type of protein that is shown to suppress appetite, Presents fullness compared to different proteins like whey, casein or soy, helps in maintaining muscles and even the presence of cellulite Helps to reduce it can improve the elasticity of the skin and thickness. For greater information at the benefits of collagen, seek advice from this newsletter, and it is a nice manner to supplement it in your weight-reduction plan.

• Greens Powder

And getting enough vitamins to support healthy weight loss and overall well-being is extremely important. Taking multivitamin in combination with synthetic materials is ineffective and shown as a complete waste of money. Alternatively, consuming high-quality greens made of real, nutritious whole foods rich in vitamins, minerals, antioxidants, fibers, and phytonutrients is a better way of optimizing health and longevity. See this article for more information about supplemented with high quality, effective greens powder.

- Probiotics

Lose gut health is extremely important for anyone to lose weight and increase overall health. This is not uncommon for those who make changes in the ketogenic diet for the change in bacterial production in their colon (although not necessarily a bad thing - just a change). To support this change and to help healthy bacteria in your intestine, try to consume supplemented with more fermented foods such as secret, kimchi or kefir and high quality probiotic.

- Vitamin D

That is anticipated that over 50% of the world's people lack vitamin D deficiency. Although vitamin D is in Ketosis, it plays a major role; it is responsible for regulating immunity, swelling, hormones, and helping with all the factors important for overall health, with electrolyte absorption. Also, studies support the direct benefits of vitamin D for weight loss. You can check the level of your vitamin D with a simple blood test, and then you can supplement accordingly. When completing, choose Vitamin D3 because it is the form that is best absorbed by your body.

• L-Glutamine

L-glutamine is an amino acid with many capabilities for your frame which acts as a powerful antioxidant. Research shows that L-glutamine can help in stabilizing blood sugar levels, which has been recommended to help reduce sugar deficiency. With the help of L-glutamine (approximately 1-1 teaspoon powder or 500 mg supplements), supplementary carb/sugar can reduce cravings and assist in your ketogenic weight loss journey.

• Bull bile

Those who had removed their gall bladder, they may need bull biliary supplementation to support their body in fat digestion. When taken with food, the bull provides a concentrated source of gall-gall which takes place in the bile, which is secreted by your gallbladder.

As mentioned earlier, proper digestion is important in helping to lose weight and optimize overall health and well-being.

Conclusion:

Thank you for making it through to Keto Meal Plan for 30 Days, let's hope it was educational and Able to supply you with all the tools that you want to realize your goals for Weight loss journey. The next step is to would be to recall the menu choices and head to the market. Pay attention to the seasons and prepare your menu on the Items which can be found fresh from the plants. Thus, a lot of the time can be saved by using Keto Kitchen Basics for cooking demands.

Deciding upon a keto meal preparation for weight loss, can help you to be healthier, think clearer, live longer, and weight loss. It takes a while to become used to it, even though there are lots of foods you may enjoy in this book that can allow this diet to feel much more like a feast.

Regardless of your age, fitness level, or the general condition of wellness, the meal prep can help you stay better. So many Individuals have attained Weight loss goals and their fitness thanks for this. It is your opportunity to create your dream body that you always want with the health you always want.